KAYCE GOODMAN

Lazy Girl Workouts

A Gym Hater's Guide to TV-time Toning

Contents

1

Introduction

Welcome, fellow gym-avoiders and exercise skeptics, to a delightful little journey I like to call 'Lazy Girl Workouts: A Gym Hater's Guide to TV-time Toning.' Now, before you roll your eyes and reach for the remote, hear me out. I'm not here to transform you into the next cover model for a fitness magazine. Far from it. I'm just like you - someone who finds the idea of sweating it out in a gym about as appealing as a root canal.

Why did I write this book? Well, it all started with a simple realization: my couch and I were in a very committed relationship, but my muscles and I, unfortunately, were not. I noticed the subtle signs of muscle loss – the slight struggle while carrying groceries, mushy-looking arms, the huffing and puffing after a flight of stairs. Sound familiar? I wanted to keep my body in decent shape without sacrificing my cherished couch-potato time after a long day of work. So, I started pressing a small medicine ball over my head while lying on the couch watching TV in the evenings. When this yielded results, and even compliments, I embarked on a mission: to find the easiest, most passive ways to stay toned everywhere while indulging in more appealing things –

like watching TV. And, in true lazy girl fashion, I utilized OpenAI's ChatGPT as a tool for brainstorming, drafting, and refining content for the creation of this book.

Inside, you'll find a treasure trove of exercises so simple, any self-respecting Lazy Girl can appreciate them. We're talking about movements that can be seamlessly integrated into your daily routine, requiring minimal effort and zero gym memberships. Imagine toning up while you're lost in the latest drama series or even during those long Zoom calls. We'll use everyday items like resistance bands, medicine balls, and light wearable weights – nothing that screams 'I'm trying too hard.'

Each chapter is designed to take you through different aspects of your at-home, TV-compatible workout journey. We start with 'Planning & Props,' where we'll dive into the essential, yet unobtrusive, equipment you'll need. Then, in 'Rehearsals,' we ease you into this new world of casual fitness. The following chapters, 'Core & Abs Day', 'Chest Up Day', and 'Butt Up Day,' focus on specific muscle groups, ensuring you cover all bases without breaking a sweat. 'Stretching & Mobility Day' will keep you limber and prevent any couch-induced stiffness. Finally, 'Sample Schedule & Progress Tracking' helps you keep track of your journey without turning it into a full-time job.

The beauty of 'Lazy Girl Workouts' lies in its simplicity and subtlety. You're not training for a marathon or prepping for a bodybuilding contest. You're simply adding a sprinkle of movement to your current daily routine to keep those muscles engaged and happy. It's about making toning so effortless, you'll hardly notice you're doing it – until you do.

So, let's embark on this journey together. By the end of this book, you'll have mastered the art of keeping fit while fully immersed in your leisure time. Who knows, you might even find yourself looking forward to these sneaky little exercises. Now, let's turn the page and step – very gently – into the world of 'Lazy Girl Workouts.'

2

Planning & Props

Alright, intrepid home exercisers, it's time to talk about the nitty-gritty: setting up your very own, ultra-comfy workout space. This isn't about creating a mini-gym (heaven forbid!). It's more like preparing your living room (or any room, really) for a little activity beyond the usual Netflix marathons.

Choosing the Ideal Workout Space

First things first, let's pick your spot. You don't need a vast, sun-drenched room with panoramic views. Just a cozy corner where you can stretch out without knocking over a lamp. You'll need two key areas: a place to sit (like your couch or a sturdy chair) and a spot to lie down (a yoga mat on the floor works wonders). Remember, the aim is to integrate exercise into your everyday life, not to turn your living room into a space that screams 'sweat and pain.'

Suggested Equipment to Have On-Hand

Now, let's talk props. No, not the heavy, intimidating types you find in gyms. Think simple, portable, and not an eyesore. These are simple, affordable tools that pack a punch without taking up space. The props outlined below are all easily storable under the couch or in a drawer. These are your new best friends, ready to add a little extra oomph to your routines without feeling like you're lugging around medieval weaponry.

Light Wearable Weights

First up, wearable wrist/ankle weights. These are perfect for adding a bit of resistance to your exercises without going overboard. You can find them at most sporting goods stores or online retailers like Amazon or Walmart. Look for weights ranging from 1 to 3 pounds – they're enough to add some challenge but not so much that you'll feel like you're training for the Olympics.

Resistance Bands

Next, let's talk about resistance bands. They're versatile, easy to store, and great for a range of exercises. Again, these can be found at most sports stores or online. When choosing, consider bands with different resistance levels – light, medium, and heavy – to mix up your workouts as you grow stronger. I recommend obtaining at least one open-ended band as well as a closed loop band. For a DIY alternative, old pantyhose or tights can be surprisingly effective. They're stretchy and durable, making them a fantastic makeshift resistance band.

Medicine Ball

A soft medicine ball is a fun addition, especially for core, chest, and shoulder exercises. These can be a bit pricier, but they last a long time and can be used in various ways. Look for one that's soft-ish and not too heavy – around 2 to 8 pounds - and small enough to hold in one hand. I got mine at the discount store Five Below, so don't be afraid to look at your local discount store for these gems. If you're feeling industrious, a garden-variety balloon filled with sand or rice is an option.

Multi-Use Yoga Mat

Lastly, a yoga mat. It's not just for yoga; it's your foundation for floor exercises and stretching. Mats provide cushioning, prevent slipping, and - in my case - keep the dog hair from coating my backside! You can find affordable options at department stores or online, but great no-cost alternatives include a thick bathroom or throw rug or a couple of layered beach towels.

Optional Bonus Items

Don't worry, nobody is grading you, but if you want to expand on your mindless fitness, don't mind the eyesore, and have the space, consider adding a hula hoop, a jump rope, and/or a stability ball to your arsenal. I'll offer a few bonus-related exercise options in Chapters 4-7 for you to incorporate or ignore as you see fit!

Remember, the goal here isn't to break the bank but to make exercising at home as easy and accessible as possible. Whether you buy new equipment or improvise with what you have, the key is to start moving. With these tools at your disposal, you're all set to turn your living space into a casual workout haven.

Setting Up Your Workout Space

Setting up your space is as easy as 1-2-3. Keep your equipment within arm's reach of your chosen workout area. This could be a small basket beside the couch or a dedicated drawer in your TV stand. I keep mine in a storage ottoman. The key is convenience – you're more likely to use something if it's right there, staring at you during your TV binges. Next, ensure your TV or laptop is in a good position – after all, you'll need to have a good view of it to distract you while you 'work out.'

Remember, your workout space doesn't have to look like it's ripped out of a fitness magazine. It should feel like a natural part of your home, a place where exercise sneaks into your routine so smoothly, you barely notice it. After all, isn't that the dream?

So there we have it! A simple, effective, and decidedly un-gym-like space for your 'Lazy Girl Workouts.' Now, we're ready to get started!

3

Rehearsals

Welcome to the heart of our 'Lazy Girl Workouts,' where we set the stage for beginning your journey safely and effectively. This chapter is your guide to using these exercises not just casually, but wisely, ensuring you reap maximum benefits without any unwanted setbacks.

Safety Basics

First and foremost, let's talk about safety. Proper form is crucial, even in these low-intensity exercises. Always keep your movements controlled and smooth. Avoid jerky or rushed motions, as they can lead to strain. Since we will be focusing on toning, remember to start light with your weights and resistance bands. We will be targeting high repetition, so what feels easy at first could wipe you out by the end. And remember, if something hurts (in a sharp, painful way, not the 'I'm working muscles I never knew I had' way), stop immediately. Pain is your body's way of saying something's not right. Listen to it and be patient with yourself.

Exercise Rotation & Tips for Consuming Upcoming Chapters

Since we aren't going for high intensity fitness here, consistency and repetition will be key. The goal is for these exercises to become a habit while allowing our minds to forget we're exercising at all! To achieve this, I suggest first trying each movement as you read through the next few chapters so you understand how to do them and how each one can fit into your version of TV time, your chosen space, and the props that you have available to you. I've included illustrations of many of them, particularly those you may not be familiar with.

Then, in Chapter 8 I'll provide some ideas for rotating through the exercises to target different muscle groups on different days of the week for maximum results. Variety keeps things fresh and prevents overworking any single muscle group. Before you know it, you'll have mastered these movements enough to mindlessly incorporate them into your leisure time.

Rest & Recovery

Rest and recovery are just as important as the exercises themselves. Your muscles need time to repair and strengthen, especially if you're new to exercising. Include rest days in your schedule, or at least days where you focus solely on light stretching or mobility work. This approach helps prevent injury and ensures your muscles have time to adapt and grow stronger.

A Word About Diet

Lastly, a quick note on diet. While this isn't a diet book, it's worth mentioning that overeating can counteract your exercise efforts. You don't necessarily need to follow a strict diet to tone your muscles, but if you want to actually see them above a healthy layer of mush, be mindful of your eating habits. Focus on nourishing your body with small balanced meals rather than restricting yourself. At the very least, consider how these exercises keep your body busy during TV-time when perhaps it used to be mindlessly shoveling snacks instead!

So there you have it – your guide to starting off on the right foot, or the left, depending on your preference. Next up, we'll delve into the how-to specifics of each exercise, grouped into major body sections, then offer a suggested schedule of how to incorporate them into your couch-time routine. Here's to beginning your journey to better health, one lazy workout at a time!

4

Core & Abs Day

In this chapter, you will learn exercises that target your core strength and abdominal toning. We'll use a variety of props like resistance bands, weights, and medicine balls to add some fun and effectiveness to your routine. Your goal will be to incorporate at least one day of core and ab work per week.

As you work through this chapter, remember to try each exercise and familiarize yourself with each movement. Ultimately, you will be asked to complete one exercise from each sub-section below on your chosen Core/Ab days, so feel free to mark your favorites in each section or even cross one out if it simply doesn't work for your body's capabilities.

Core Strength Exercises (*Try all; pick one on Core/Ab Days*)

A strong core is essential for just about everything, from maintaining good posture to preventing injuries. Strengthening your core is like giving your body a solid foundation. It's not just about getting a toned belly; it's about improving balance, stability, and overall well being. Let's explore some core exercises that are perfect for doing during

TV time, incorporating balance and cleverly timed with your chosen entertainment.

Planks

- Exercise: Get into a plank position on your elbows and toes. Some might prefer to be on hands and toes, which is ok too. Keep your body in a straight line, engaging your core muscles. Try these in front of a full length mirror until you memorize the body position.
- Timing Tip: Start holding the plank during a commercial break. Aim for 30 seconds at a time and gradually increase the duration as you grow stronger. As your strength improves, challenge yourself to hold it for an entire commercial segment. Repeat during each commercial segment of a TV show. Be creative if your chosen entertainment doesn't come with commercial breaks. A timer on your phone or simply counting will work too.

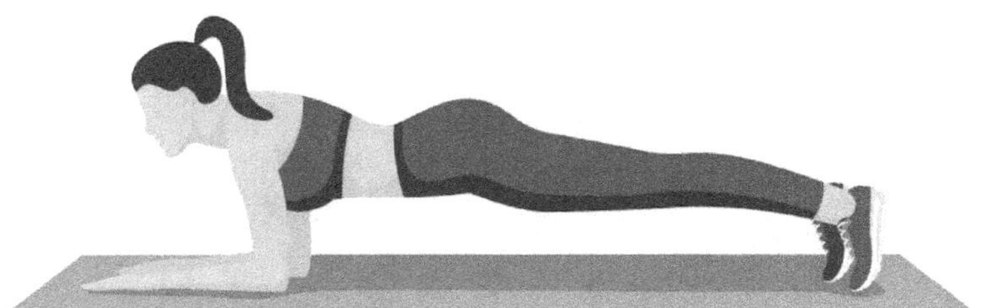

Seated Twists

- Exercise: Sit on the floor or on your couch with legs bent, lean back slightly without rounding your back, and twist your torso from side to side. Optionally, hold a lightweight object like a medicine ball for added resistance. Be sure to twist slowly and methodically to avoid back strain.
- Timing Tip: Do this 20 times, 10 on each side, at a time then rest. Aim to repeat this 5 to 10 times throughout your show, completing a total of 50 to 100 per side. Remember to listen to your body and work your way to your goal over time.

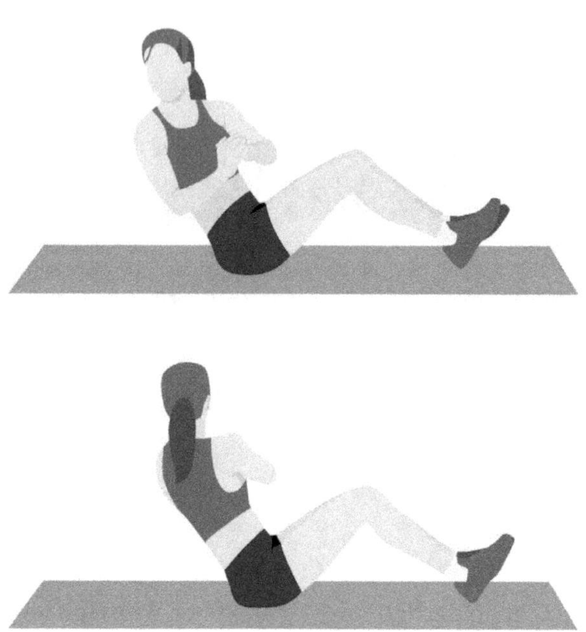

Balancing Leg Lifts

- Exercise: Stand behind your couch or a chair for support. Lift one leg to the side and hold it for a few seconds, then switch legs. This not only works your core but also improves balance, especially the less you rely on that chair or couch for stability. If side leg lifting is difficult, try standing on one leg like a flamingo instead. When you feel shaky, remember to tighten your core and abs!
- Timing Tip: Perform this exercise during dialogue-heavy scenes. Balance on one leg while a character speaks, then switch legs when the next character starts talking. If you are watching sports, use

team possession changes as your leg-changing signal instead. Rest as needed.

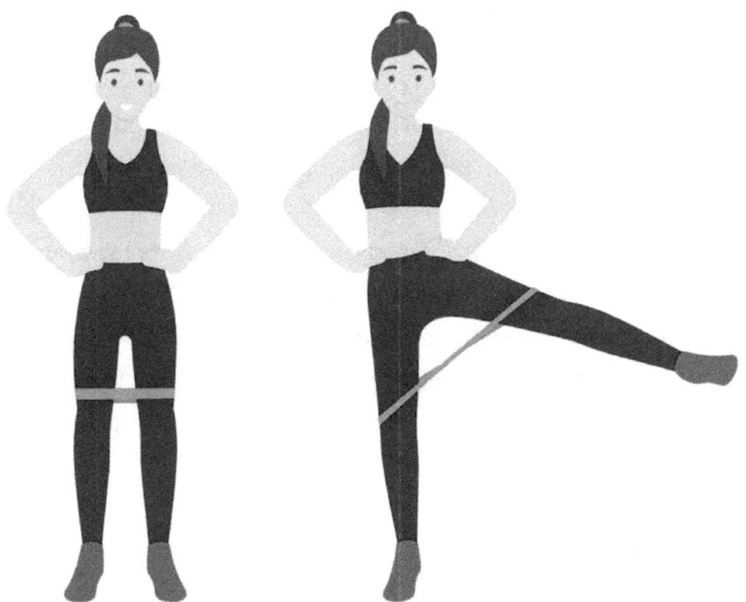

Bonus: Stability Ball Sits

- Exercise: If you have a stability ball, try sitting on it instead of the couch. It forces you to engage your core to maintain balance while you watch TV. This is an easy alternative to the balancing leg lifts for those extra-lazy days!
- Timing Tip: Use the ball during your favorite show or a movie. The

longer the program, the more time you spend engaging those core muscles.

Abdominal Exercises (*Try all; pick one on Core/Ab Days*)

Specifically targeting the abdominals not only enhances your core strength, but can uncover a waist and more toned belly that may have become illusive in recent years! Here are some easy and effective abdominal exercises to get familiar with. We will be coupling one abdominal exercise with a core exercise from above on Core/Ab days so go ahead and rehearse each of them!

Timing Tip: Plan to incorporate these ab exercises into the timing of the core exercise you've chosen to couple with them. For example, if you are working during commercial breaks, do your core exercise during the first half of the show and your ab exercise during the second half. Experiment and find what works for you, but be sure you are working your way toward a high repetition of each on a given day.

Lying Leg Lifts

- Exercise: Lie on your back with your legs straight. Slowly raise them up to the ceiling and then lower them back down without touching the floor. This is great for your lower abs. If you need lower back support like me, place your hands or a rolled up towel under your lower back or tailbone for support, or modify the movement by bringing your knees to your chest in a reverse crunch instead. Finally, hooking your hands under the couch above your head can provide added stability.
- Repetitions: Start with 10 lifts at a time with a resting minute or

two in between. Increase how many you do at a time as you get stronger.

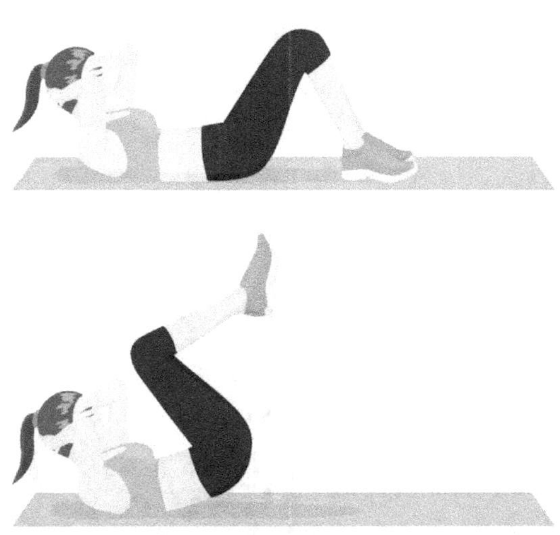

Bicycle Crunches

- Exercise: Lie on your back, place your hands behind your head, and alternate bringing your elbow and opposite knee together, mimicking a cycling motion.
- Repetitions: Start with 20 touches (10 on each side) at a time, then rest. Aim to repeat this 5 to 10 times throughout your show, completing a total of 50 to 100 per side. Remember to listen to your body and work your way to your goal over time.

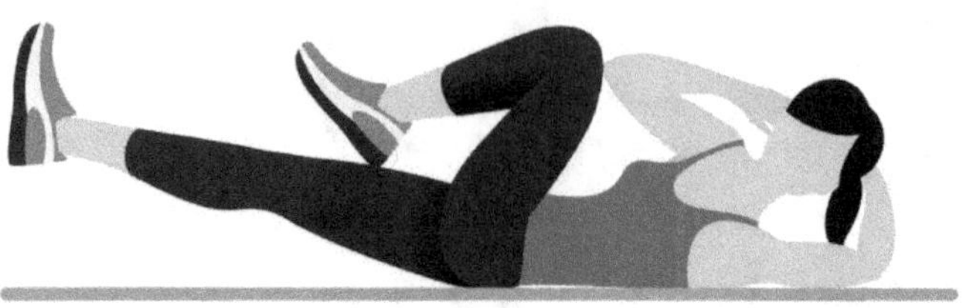

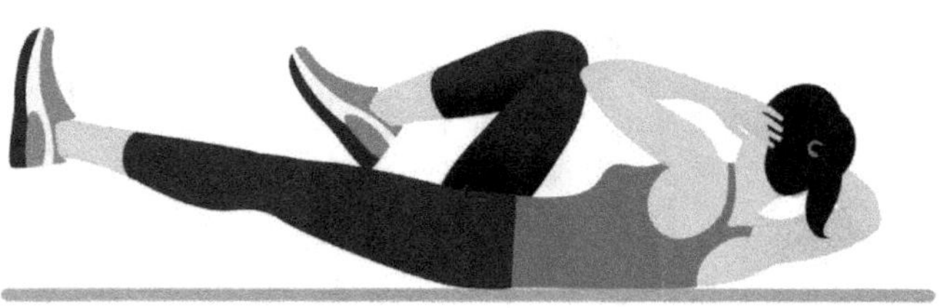

Pilates Hundred

- Exercise: Lie on your back with your hands by your sides, palms down. Raise your legs to a 45-degree angle, lift your head and shoulders, and hold that position as you rapidly pump your arms up and down in a small fluttering motion.
- Repetitions: Work in sets of 20 arm pumps at a time using your breathing to pace yourself (inhale for 5 pumps, exhale for 5 pumps, inhale for 5 pumps, exhale for 5 pumps, rest and repeat). As you gain strength, try increasing to 40 pumps at a time and so forth up to 100. If counting while consuming your favorite movie or show

is difficult, use a phone timer or a show-related trigger to challenge yourself instead.

Bonus: Hula Hooping

- Exercise: If you have a hula hoop and enough space, try reconnecting with your younger self with a few minutes of sustained hooping! Sure it isn't a couch-worthy exercise, but it is fun and great for your core, abs, and mobility. If you are like me, you'll be rusty at first so keep trying and celebrate those small victories as you progress!
- Timing Tip: Try this during a music montage in your programming to help you keep rhythm.

By syncing these abdominal exercises with different parts of your TV shows or movies, you create a fun and engaging way to work on your core strength and abdominal toning. It's all about making the most of your leisure time by adding a twist of health and fitness.

5

'Chest Up' Day

This chapter is all about producing results from your chest, up! The following exercises cover biceps, triceps, shoulders, chest, and back, all without breaking a sweat. For simplicity, I've broken this chapter into three sub-sections: Arm Toning where you will aim to do all three exercises, and Chest Toning and Back Toning where you will aim to do one of each.

Arm Toning Exercises (*Do all on Chest Up Days*)

Toning your arms can be a simple, yet effective part of your at-home workout, especially when you pair it with your entertainment schedule. Using a medicine ball or resistance band, we can target the biceps, triceps, and shoulders in the same day with exercises that are easy to do from your couch or in front of your favorite distraction. Here's how:

Bicep Curls

- Exercise: While sitting on the edge of the couch or a chair or while standing, trap the middle of a resistance band securely under your feet and grasp the other end of the band in each hand. Starting with your hands down by your side, curl your palms up towards your shoulders while keeping your elbows stationary and close to your body at the waist. You can also alternate arms if you prefer.

- Repetitions: Aim for 10-15 curls per arm before resting. Work in sets each week until you are able to complete a total of 50 or more per arm each session. Remember, if counting while consuming your favorite movie or show is too distracting, use a phone timer or a show-related trigger to pace yourself instead.

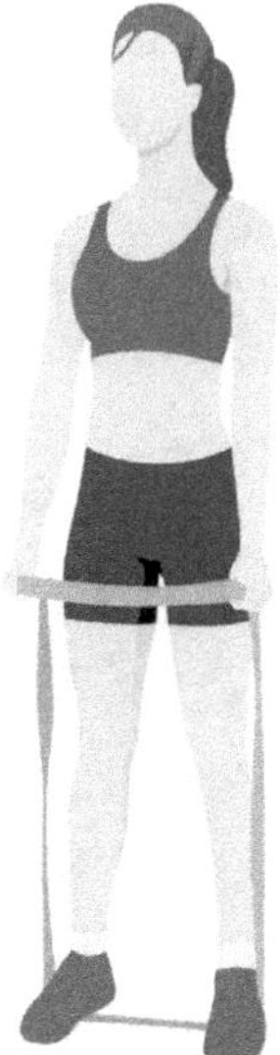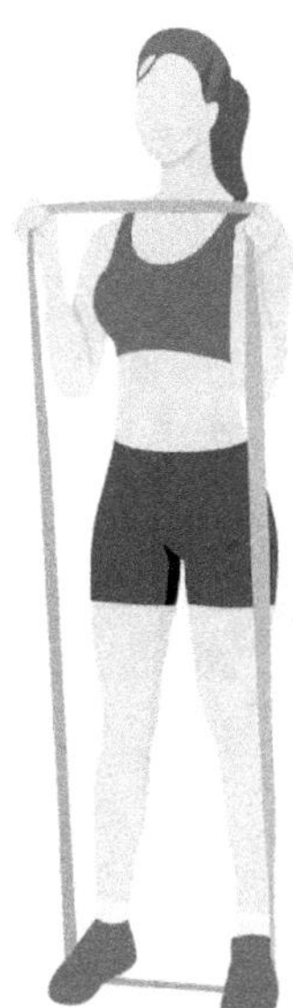

Tricep Extensions

- Exercise: Either stand firmly on the center of your open-ended resistance band and grasp one end of the band in each hand or hold one end of a folded band in each hand. Starting with one hand stationary in front of you, extend the other behind you 45 degrees, keeping your arm straight. Switch sides and repeat by extending the opposite arm. If you need additional resistance, choke down on the band or use a shorter or thicker band. This exercise can be modified by using a light dumbbell or attaching wearable weights to each wrist.
- Repetitions: Start with 10-15 extensions per arm before resting. Work in sets of 10 or more each week until you are able to complete a total of 50 or more per arm each time.

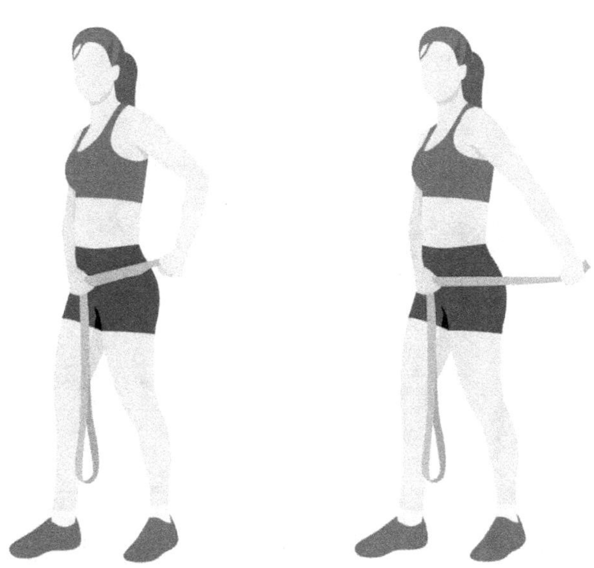

Shoulder Press

- Exercise: Sit or stand with erect posture and with a medicine ball in one hand. Start with the ball at shoulder level similar to a waiter holding a tray. Slowly push the ball up over your head, extending your arm fully, then slowly lower it back down to starting position.
- Repetitions: Do 10 presses with one arm before switching to the other to complete the set. Work toward 5 sets of 20 per arm, resting in between sets, and you'll be pressing 100 times an arm before you know it!

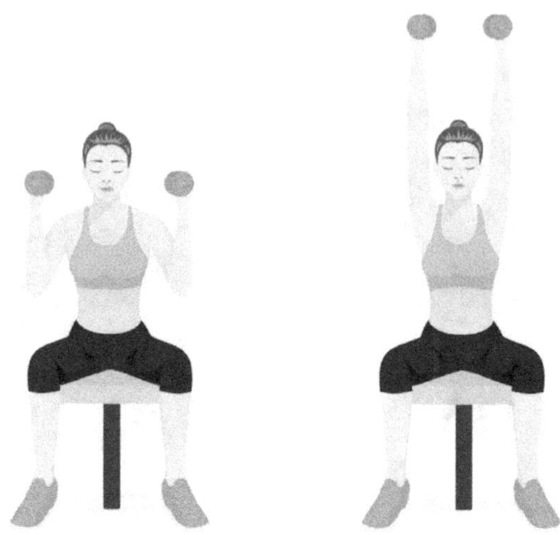

Chest Toning Exercises (*Try all; pick one on Chest Up Days*)

Too frequently, we ladies ignore chest toning because we aren't really in the 'big pecks' business. However, toned pectoral muscles can help support the business we do have going on there!

Ideally, you'll choose one of the following to pair with the above arm toning exercises on the same day, but if time doesn't allow for it, choose one of these and pair it with one of the back exercises on a separate day.

Chest Press with Resistance Band

- Exercise: While seated or lying down, wrap a resistance band around your back and hold the ends in each hand. Press your hands forward as if you're pushing against a wall, then relax. If there is too much slack in the band to feel any resistance, change your hand position on the band.

- Repetitions: Do 10 presses with one arm before switching to the other to complete the set. Work toward 5 sets of 20 per arm, resting in between sets.

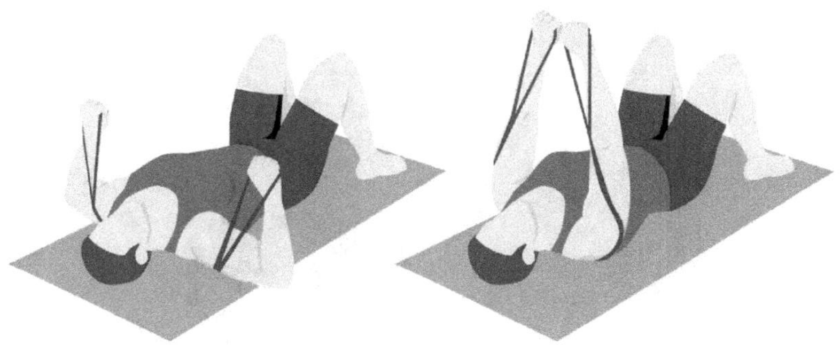

Medicine Ball Chest Press

This is my personal favorite and where the Lazy Girl Workout began! I do 100 of these on each arm, 20 at a time, with an 8 lb medicine ball. As a bonus, it works those triceps too!

- Exercise: Lie flat on your back with your knees bent. Hold your medicine ball in one hand near your collarbone, elbow at your waist. To begin, extend your arm straight up toward the ceiling, then lower it back down. Be sure to use smooth controlled movement.
- Repetitions: Start with 10 presses with each hand, followed by a brief rest. Work toward 5 sets of 20 per arm as you grow stronger.

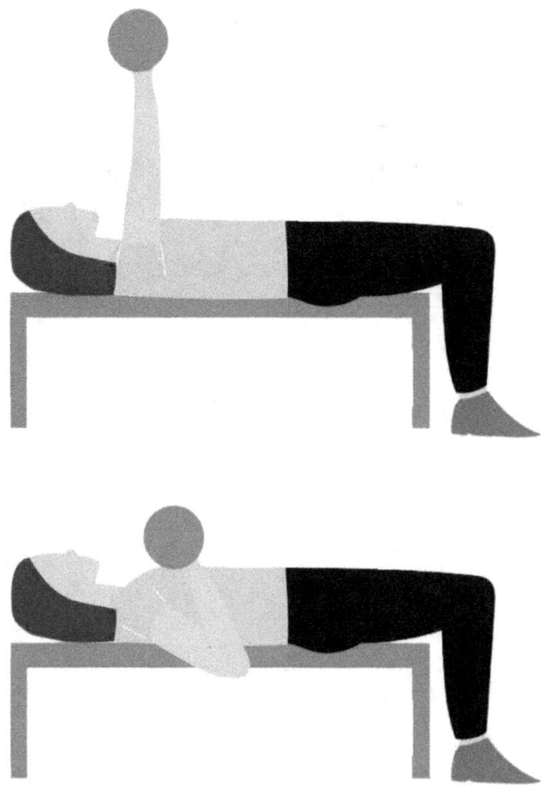

Back Toning Exercises (*Try all; pick one on Chest Up Days*)

Bent-Over Rows with Resistance Band

- Exercise: Stand on the middle of an open-ended resistance band, holding the ends in each hand. Bend your knees slightly, hinging forward at your waist, hands resting near the outside of each knee and palms facing up. Using both hands at the same time, pull the band up towards your waist, bending your arms at the elbow and squeezing your back muscles as your shoulder blades move toward each other.
- Repetitions: Start with sets of 10-15 rows and gradually work up to 100 total rows per session over time.

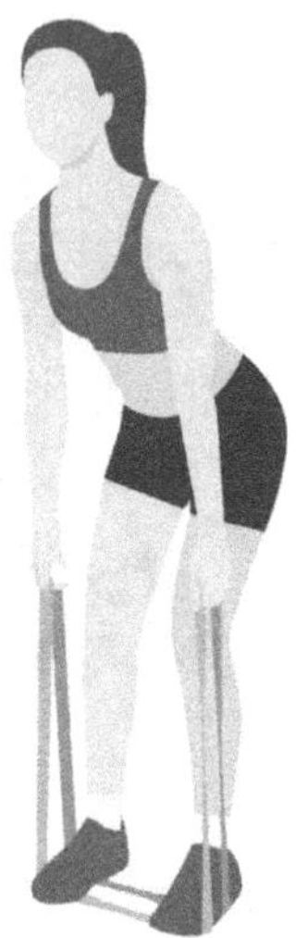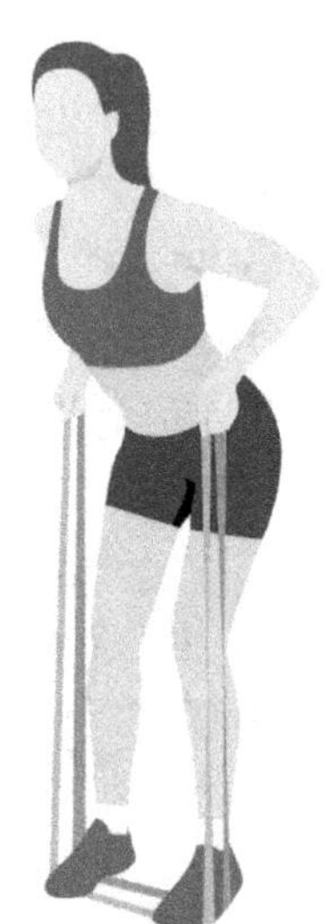

Resistance Band Chest Stretch

- Exercise: Hold a resistance band straight out in front of you at chest level. To begin, pull your arms out to opposing sides, opening up your chest and squeezing your shoulder blades together.
- Repetitions: Hold each stretch for 10-15 seconds. Repeat as many times as you can during a segment of your TV show, like the opening or closing credits.

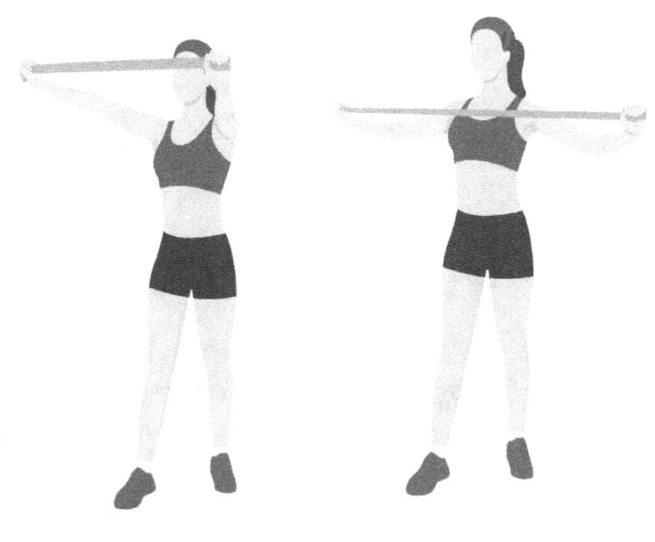

By incorporating these exercises into your TV routine, you'll be enhancing your upper body strength and tone, all while keeping up with your favorite series. Remember, the key is consistent repetition without the posturing and grunting. Your living room is now your gym, and your favorite show is the perfect workout partner!

6

'Butt Up' Day

Ok, to be fair, we will really be working next on our butts and everything *below* - but let's face it - what girl doesn't want to keep her butt more *up*?! So as we continue our journey of 'Lazy Girl Workouts,' it's time to focus on the lower body. Toning the legs and buttocks not only improves appearance but also enhances overall strength and stability. As with the previous chapters, we'll use a mix of simple tools like resistance bands, light weights, and balance exercises to work those lower body muscles from the comfort of your living room.

On these Butt Up days, you'll want to work one exercise from each subsection below for full effect. So go ahead and learn them all and then rotate one each into your Butt Up days according to your preference.

Butt Toning Exercises (*Try all; pick one on Butt Up Days*)

Squats with Resistance Band

- Exercise: Stand with your feet shoulder-width apart, a resistance

30

band looped around your thighs. Squat down as if sitting in a chair, keeping your weight in your heels. If you are worried about your balance, be sure the couch is behind you for a soft landing!

- Repetitions: Aim for 15-20 squats at a time, then rest and repeat every few minutes. Build up to five rounds or more.
- Timing Tip: Do this during a show's first scene and every scene coming out of a commercial break, for example, to keep your mind off the effort.

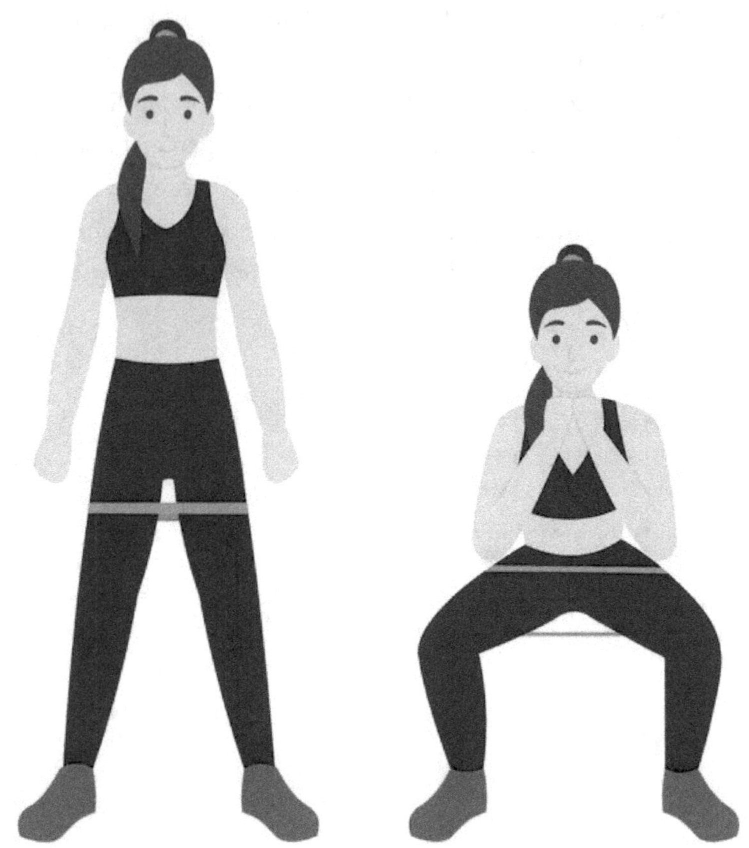

Glute Bridges

- Exercise: Lie on your back with your hands by your side, your knees bent, and feet flat on the floor. Lift your hips towards the ceiling, squeezing your glutes at the top. If this creates discomfort in your neck, try adding a small pillow to support it.
- Repetitions: Perform 20 bridges at a time. Pause at the top of the last one for as long as you can. Rest then repeat up to five times. As you grow stronger, consider adding extra resistance by resting

your wearable weights across your lower abdomen.

- Timing Tip: Use the more relaxed, slower-paced segments of your show for this exercise, focusing on your form and the contraction of your glute muscles.

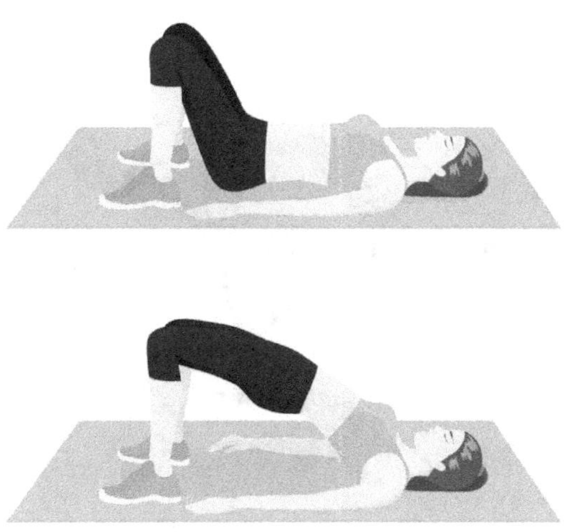

Donkey Kicks with Resistance Band

- Exercise: Get on all fours with a looped resistance band around one foot and anchored under your hands (or the opposite ankle) at the other side. Kick the banded leg back and up, focusing on squeezing your glutes.
- Repetitions: Start out with 10 kicks on each side until you are comfortable with the movement. Increase repetitions when you are able and work up to at least five sets of kicks per leg.

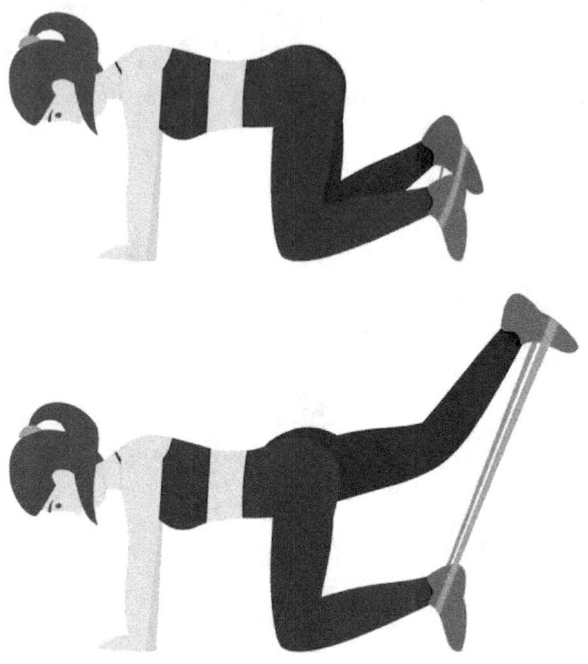

Side Leg Raises

- Exercise: Lie on your side, knees bent or straight, and legs stacked. Support your head with a pillow or your hand or prop yourself up on one elbow. Lift the upper leg to about 45 degrees then lower it back down using slow, controlled motions. Be sure not to roll your body back or forward during this movement. Aim to remain perpendicular to the floor. Over time, consider adding a looped resistance band around both legs just above the knees. Only do this as your strength permits.
- Repetitions: Aspire to perform 20 raises five times on each side for

a total of 100 per leg.

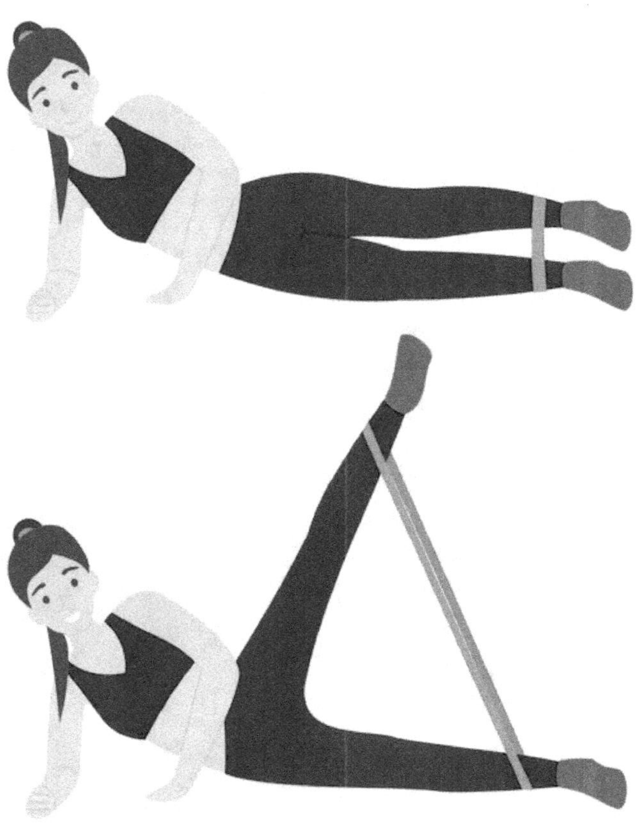

Quadriceps and Hamstrings Exercises (*Try all; pick one on Butt Up Days*)

Lunges with Light Weights

- Exercise: Holding light weights or a medicine ball in front of you, step forward into a lunge, keeping your front knee over your ankle and pressing your back knee toward the floor. Then push off your front leg and back to the starting position. Alternate legs. Use the couch or a chair for stability if needed and only until you are strong enough to do these without it.

• Repetitions: Start with 10 lunges on each leg and work your way up to more as you progress each week. Rest and repeat this 5 times.

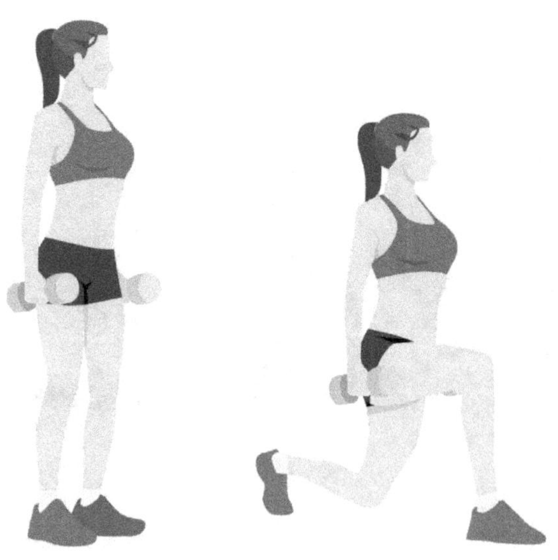

Standing Leg Extensions & Butt Kicks

- Exercise: Wearing your ankle weights, stand near a chair or couch back for balance as needed. Extend one leg straight in front of you to between 45 and 90 degrees according to your ability and comfort level, then lower it back down. Then take your foot on the same leg and bend it toward your behind, keeping your knees parallel. Both motions together count as one repetition. Repeat both motions on each leg.
- Repetitions: Do 10-20 extension-butt kick combinations per leg. Rest and aim to repeat for five sets of 10-20 on each leg. It does not matter if you alternate legs each repetition or complete one leg before moving to the other.

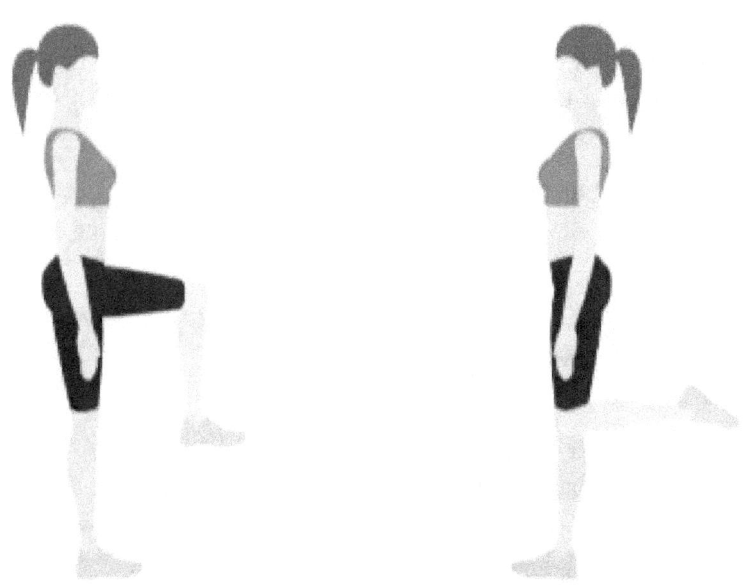

Calf and Shin Exercises (*Try all; pick one on Butt Up Days*)

Calf Raises Seated or Standing

- Exercise: Stand with your feet hip-width apart. Raise up onto your tiptoes and then lower back down. Use a chair or couch back for stability if needed. If you prefer, these can also be done seated on a chair or the couch with your feet on the floor and weights resting on your knees for some resistance.
- Repetitions: Complete 20-25 calf raises at a time. Rest and repeat five times.

Seated Toe Taps

- Exercise: Sitting on a chair or the couch with your feet flat on the floor, lift your toes up and down, leaving your heels on the floor throughout the movement.
- Repetitions: Do this for about 1 minute, then rest for 1 minute. Repeat 5 times.
- Timing Tip: Ideal for moments in your show where you need to pay more attention to the plot, as it requires little focus on the exercise itself.

Resistance Band Ankle Flexions

- Exercise: Sit with your legs straight out in front of you and loop a resistance band around the balls of your feet. Holding the other end(s) of the band, slowly point and flex your feet against the resistance, working the calf and shin muscles.
- Repetitions: Do this for about 1 minute, then rest for 1 minute. Repeat 5 times.

Bonus: Jumping Rope

- Exercise: If you have a jump rope and enough space, try jumping rope for added intensity. I know this will get your blood pumping beyond Lazy Girl levels, but it is fun, will burn a few extra calories, and works your whole lower body at once!
- Timing Tip: Try this during a music montage or during commercial breaks so you won't have to crank the volume over your huffing and puffing.

By integrating these lower body exercises into your routine, you'll not only tone your legs and booty, but also enhance your overall body strength and stability. Remember, it's about consistency and mindless repetition, so no need to dread leg day when doing it the Lazy Girl way!

7

Stretching & Mobility Day

As we gracefully mature, you may notice it seems like everything hurts. This is partially because our bodies crave more attention in the form of stretching and mobility work. It's not just about keeping muscles beautifully elongated; it's about maintaining the range of motion, reducing the risk of injury, and enhancing overall quality and fluidity of movement.

This chapter will guide you through various stretching and mobility exercises that you will use on your "rest" days to ensure that you stay limber and agile. Daily stretching is always beneficial, but aim to do each of these exercises at least once a week.

Lower Body Stretching Exercises (*Do all each time*)

Ankle Circles

- Exercise: Sit comfortably and extend one leg. Rotate your ankle slowly, making large circles. Switch directions after a few rotations.
- Repetitions: Do 10 circles in each direction per ankle. Repeat 2-3

times.

Butterfly Stretch

- Exercise: Sit on the floor, bring the soles of your feet together, pull your feet as close to your torso as comfortably possible, and let your knees fall to the sides. Gently press your knees down with your hands or elbows for a deeper stretch.
- Repetitions: Hold the stretch for 20-30 seconds at a time, breathing deeply as you hold it. Repeat 3-5 times, resting in between. Note your increased flexibility over time as your knees get closer to the floor.

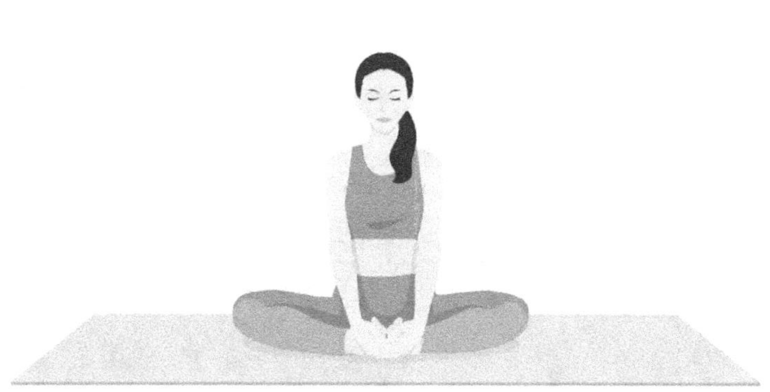

Hip Flexor Stretch

- Exercise: Kneel on one knee with the opposite foot on the floor in front of you. If needed, put a cushion under your knee for comfort. Lean forward, gently shifting your weight to the front foot, stretching the front of your hip on the other leg.
- Repetitions: Hold for 20-30 seconds on each side.

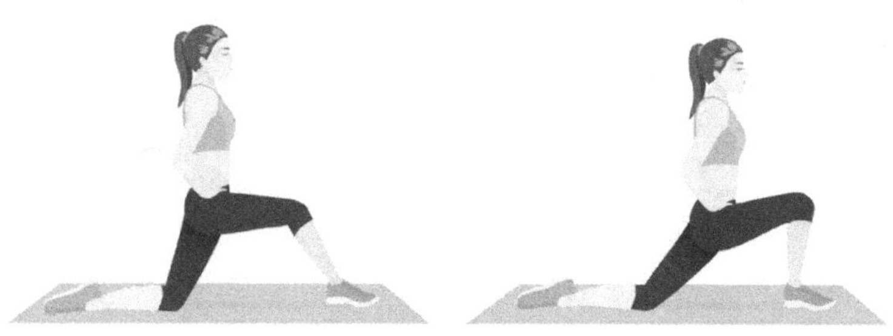

Upper Body Stretching Exercises (*Do all each time*)

Neck Tilts

- Exercise: Sit or stand comfortably. Gently tilt your head to one side, bringing your ear closer to your shoulder, and then switch sides. When finished, repeat the motion front and back, lowering your chin toward your chest first, then gently tilting it back as you look toward the ceiling.

- Repetitions: Hold each tilt for 10-15 seconds per direction. Repeat as desired.

Shoulder Rolls

- Exercise: Raise your shoulders up towards your ears, then roll them back and down in a circular motion. Once complete, change direction and roll them forward using a circular motion.
- Repetitions: Do 10-15 rolls forward and back.

Wrist Flex and Extend

- Exercise: Extend one arm in front of you, palm facing up. Gently pull back on your fingers from underneath using your other hand. Next, turn your palm facing down and repeat the same motion, using your other hand to pull your fingers under and stretch the top side of your wrist.
- Repetitions: Hold each stretch for 10-15 seconds per wrist.

Incorporating these stretching and mobility exercises into your daily routine will greatly benefit your body's flexibility and movement, especially as you age. It's a gentle yet effective way to keep your joints happy and your muscles relaxed, all while enjoying your favorite Lazy Girl activity.

Now that you've rehearsed each movement and noted those that you may not be able to do as well as your favorites, it's time to get moving with a new leisure-time toning routine!

8

Sample Schedule & Progress Tracking

C reating a habit of these low intensity exercises is crucial if you want to notice results in your strength and muscle tone. Having a structured rotation schedule and tracking your progress can significantly help. This chapter provides a sample 4-week schedule, rotating the exercises we've covered, along with a tracking template so you can see how you improve over time (in case you don't have a mirror!). Remember, the goal is to work these exercises into your favorite leisure-time activity, making it easy to be consistent, so make adjustments as needed to fit your lifestyle. I've also included a blank version for you to use when setting your own rotation schedule.

Sample Schedule of Rotation

	Week 1	Week 2	Week 3	Week 4
Monday	(Chapter 4) Core: Planks Abs: Lying Leg Lifts	(Chapter 5) Bicep Curls Tricep Extensions Shoulder Press Chest Press- Med Ball Chest Stretch w/Band	(Chapter 6) Butt: Donkey Kicks Quads/Hams: Lunges Calves: Ankle Flexions	(Chapter 7) Rest/Stretch/Mobility Ankle Circles Butterfly Stretch Hip Flexor Stretch Neck Tilts Shoulder Rolls Wrist Flex/Extend
Tuesday	(Chapter 5) Bicep Curls Tricep Extensions Shoulder Press Chest Press- Resistance Band Bent-Over Rows w/Band	(Chapter 6) Butt: Glute Bridges Quads/Hams: Lunges Calves: Toe Taps	(Chapter 7) Rest/Stretch/Mobility Ankle Circles Butterfly Stretch Hip Flexor Stretch Neck Tilts Shoulder Rolls Wrist Flex/Extend	(Chapter 4) Core: Stability Ball Sits Abs: Hula Hooping
Wednesday	(Chapter 6) Butt: Squats w/Band Quads/Hams: Leg Ext & Butt Kicks Calves: Calf Raises	(Chapter 7) Rest/Stretch/Mobility Ankle Circles Butterfly Stretch Hip Flexor Stretch Neck Tilts Shoulder Rolls Wrist Flex/Extend	(Chapter 4) Core: Balancing Leg Lifts Abs: Pilates Hundred	(Chapter 5) Bicep Curls Tricep Extensions Shoulder Press Chest Press- Med Ball Chest Stretch w/Band
Thursday	(Chapter 7) Rest/Stretch/Mobility Ankle Circles Butterfly Stretch Hip Flexor Stretch Neck Tilts Shoulder Rolls Wrist Flex/Extend	(Chapter 4) Core: Seated Twists Abs: Bicycle Crunches	(Chapter 5) Bicep Curls Tricep Extensions Shoulder Press Chest Press- Resistance Band Bent-Over Rows w/Band	(Chapter 6) Butt: Side Leg Raises Quads/Hams: Leg Ext & Butt Kicks Calves: Calf Raises
Friday	(Chapter 4) Core: Planks Abs: Lying Leg Lifts	(Chapter 5) Bicep Curls Tricep Extensions Shoulder Press Chest Press- Med Ball Chest Stretch w/Band	(Chapter 6) Butt: Donkey Kicks Quads/Hams: Lunges Calves: Ankle Flexions	(Chapter 7) Rest/Stretch/Mobility Ankle Circles Butterfly Stretch Hip Flexor Stretch Neck Tilts Shoulder Rolls Wrist Flex/Extend
Saturday	Repeat make up a day from the week.	Repeat make up a day from the week.	Repeat make up a day from the week.	Repeat make up a day from the week.
Sunday	Repeat make up a day from the week.	Repeat make up a day from the week.	Repeat make up a day from the week.	Repeat make up a day from the week.

Schedule Rotation Template

	Week 1	Week 2	Week 3	Week 4
Monday				
Tuesday				
Wednesday				
Thursday				
Friday				
Saturday				
Sunday				

Progress Tracking

Although not required, noting repetitions, resistance used, number of sets, and/or amount of time you achieved with each movement will help you see your improvements over time and help motivate you to reach your goals. You don't have to note every time you do an exercise, just the times you improved upon the last entry for that exercise. Use notes to log any feelings or modifications, and remember to listen to your body and adjust as needed. I've provided a sample tracking format for you below.

	Sets, Reps/Time, Props	Sets, Reps/Time, Props	Sets, Reps/Time, Props	Sets, Reps/Time, Props	Notes
Core/Abs					
Planks (Sample)	3 sets of 10 sec hold	3 sets of 15 sec hold	4 sets of 15 sec hold		Did on hands, not elbows
Seated Twists (Sample)	2 sets of 20, no prop	3 sets of 20, no prop	3 sets of 20, 3# ball		

Sample Progress Tracking Method

	Sets, Reps/Time, Props	Sets, Reps/Time, Props	Sets, Reps/Time, Props	Sets, Reps/Time, Props	Notes
Core/Abs					
Planks					
Seated Twists					
Balancing Leg Lifts					
Ball Sits					
Lying Leg Lifts					
Bicycle Crunches					
Pilates 100					
Hula Hooping					

Core & Ab Tracking

	Sets, Reps/Time, Props	Sets, Reps/Time, Props	Sets, Reps/Time, Props	Sets, Reps/Time, Props	Notes
Chest Up					
Bicep Curls					
Tricep Ext			48		
Shoulder Press					
Chest Press-Ball					
Chest Press-Band					
Bent-Over Rows					
Chest Stretch					

Chest Up Tracking

	Sets, Reps/Time, Props	Sets, Reps/Time, Props	Sets, Reps/Time, Props	Sets, Reps/Time, Props	Notes
Butt Up					
Squats					
Glute Bridges			49		
Donkey Kicks					
Side Leg Raises					
Lunges					
Leg Ext/Butt Kicks					
Calf Raises					
Toe Taps					
Ankle Flexions					
Jump Rope					

Butt Up Tracking

9

Conclusion

So there you have it for 'Lazy Girl Workouts: A Gym Hater's Guide to TV-time Toning'. As we wrap up, I hope you've found a new, sustainable way to integrate casual fitness into your daily life. Remember, the beauty of these workouts lies in their adaptability. Whether you're in your twenties or enjoying the golden years, whether you're a fitness newbie or someone rediscovering their need for exercise, these workouts can be tailored to your age, limitations, and fitness level.

The key to success with these exercises is consistency. It's not about intense, sporadic sessions but rather about regular, gentle activities that can be seamlessly blended into your routine. Every small step counts, and each little effort contributes to a stronger, healthier you. The goal isn't to transform overnight but to build sustainable habits that keep your body active and toned as you enjoy the things you love – like watching your favorite TV shows.

Remember, your journey doesn't end here. This book is just the beginning. Keep experimenting with the exercises, mix and match them to keep things interesting, and most importantly, listen to your body. If something feels good, keep at it. If you encounter discomfort or pain, pull back and adjust. Your body is your best guide.

I encourage you to share your experiences with your 'Lazy Girl Workouts.' If you've enjoyed this book, found it helpful, or have suggestions for others embarking on this journey, please leave a review on Amazon. Your feedback not only supports me but also helps others find a path to fitness that breaks free from the conventional, often intimidating gym culture.

Thank you for joining me on this journey. Here's to staying fit, one TV binge session at a time!

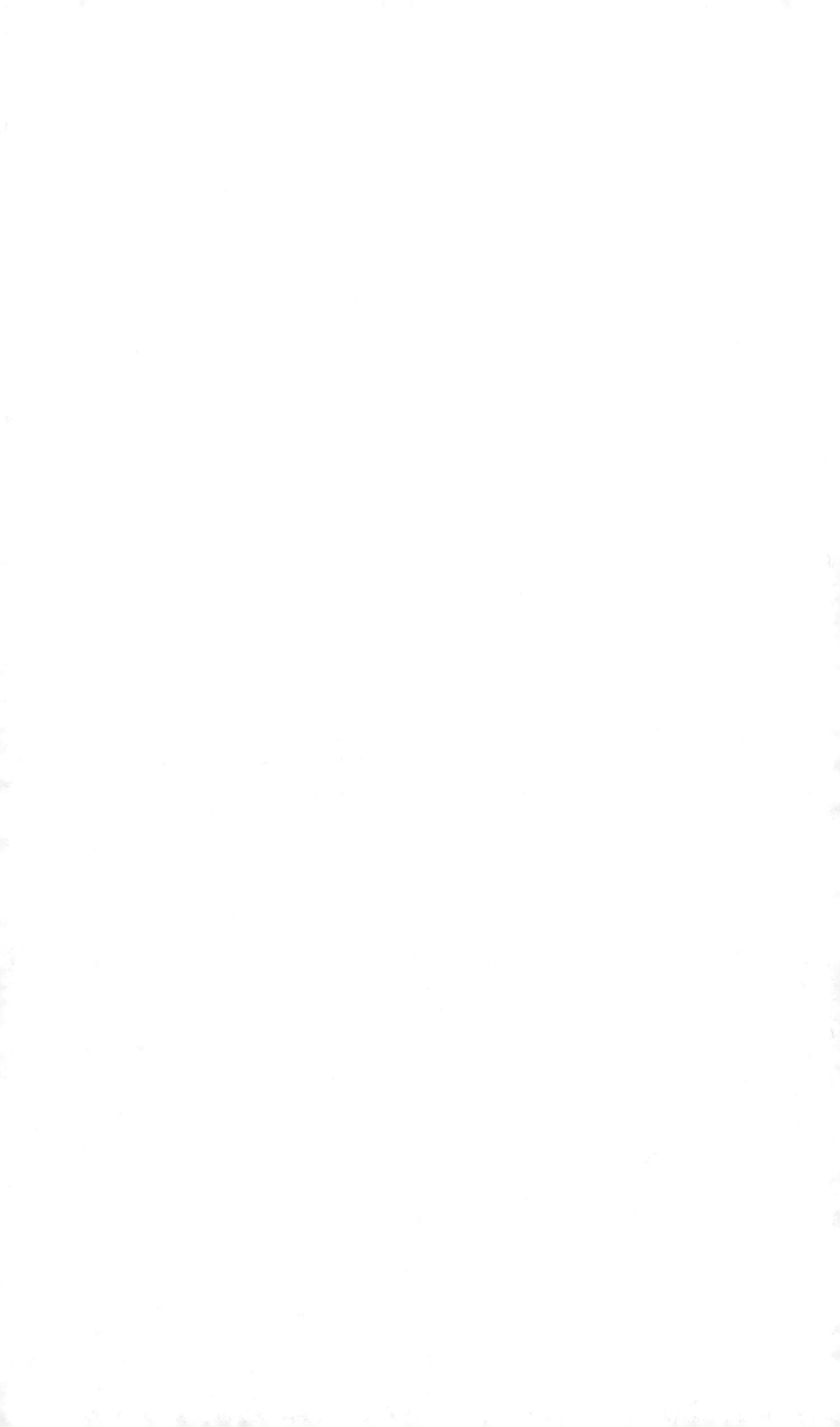